# THE DIALYSIS PROJECT

A PLAY BY

# LEAH LEWIS

WITH

# EVALYN PARRY & ROBERT CHAFE

BREAKWATER
P.O. Box 2188, St. John's, NL, Canada, A1C 6E6
WWW.BREAKWATERBOOKS.COM

COPYRIGHT © 2023 Leah Lewis
ISBN 978-1-55081-961-8

A CIP catalogue record for this book is available from Library and Archives Canada.

Cover illustration: Vanessa Iddon (Perfect Day)
Dramatic series editor: Robert Chafe

We acknowledge the support of the Canada Council for the Arts.
We acknowledge the financial support of the Government of Canada through
the Department of Heritage and the Government of Newfoundland and
Labrador through the Department of Tourism, Culture, Arts and Recreation
for our publishing activities.

PRINTED AND BOUND IN CANADA.

Canada Council   Conseil des arts   Canada    Newfoundland
for the Arts      du Canada                    Labrador

Breakwater Books is committed to choosing papers and materials for our
books that help to protect our environment. To this end, this book is printed
on recycled paper that is certified by the Forest Stewardship Council®.

This play is dedicated to
all dialysis patients and
to the nurses who support them.

# INTRODUCTION

This show went through many stages of development and public workshop presentations over the five years before its premiere, from Mount Pearl to Toronto and back. We pulled it apart and built it back up again, many times, each an attempt to capture the truth of Leah's relationship with dialysis, her machine, her body, the medical system. The truth is that the truth kept shifting, because it is complex, evolving, with tendrils of implication and resonance in all facets of Leah's life. As a creative team, we wanted to be responsive to that. We wanted *The Dialysis Project* to be nothing if not completely true to Leah at each moment of its public sharing. The version you read here is a very different version than it was even a year before it premiered. Back then we were discussing how to exemplify the solitude of Leah's dialysis experience in a public format: on stage in front of a hundred or more people. We talked about putting her on a riser out of people's reach, of hiding her in a box and making her visible only via live video feed. The ideas were never quite right, and sometimes comically wrong. But with the challenges of public health lockdowns came a somewhat imposed solution: what if Leah does her home dialysis ACTUALLY from home. The idea was so perfect it amazed us we hadn't considered it before.

Over the course of its development, versions of this show have been about disconnect, distance, tethering, crisis, fear. This incarnation still holds parts of those conversations, but in the premiere it was mostly the idea of connection that resonated throughout the show. It's deeply fitting. For the few weeks of rehearsal and production, we found ourselves masked and distanced in Leah's home, with collaborators hooked up online from Montreal, Toronto, and Charlottetown, Prince Edward Island. Leah's living room looked more like a tech booth, with lighting boards and boom mics and computers buzzing with cursors magically being commanded by designers a thousand kilometres away, in a process that wouldn't have been possible even a few short years before. It was stunning to watch. We remain deeply grateful for the expertise of the team, for their commitment to Leah and her story and for being so present though some were so far away

And we are still so grateful for the unwavering support of the staff of Resource Centre for the Arts Theatre. Thank you for making *The Dialysis Project* a reality.

Leah Lewis
Robert Chafe
Evalyn Parry

# THE DIALYSIS PROJECT

*The Dialysis Project* premiered in a livestream with Resource Centre for the Arts in St. John's, Newfoundland and Labrador, on May 25, 2021. The cast and crew were as follows.

Performed by *Leah Lewis*

Director  *Evalyn Parry*
Dramaturgy  *Robert Chafe*
Project Design Collaborator  *Kaitlin Hickey*
Lighting and Sound Design and
       Technical Direction  *Brian Kenny*
Projection Design  *Elysha Poirier*
Stage Manager  *Jana Gillis*
Livestream Technician and Camera Operator  *Emma Pope*
Puppet Design and Construction  *Kevin Woolridge*
Audience Support  *Ian Campbell*

*Ten minutes before the live feed / show begins, the screen shows a static shot of a medical table, shot from directly above. Over the course of ten minutes, we watch the table slowly getting set up with supplies for a dialysis treatment.* LEAH's *hands are seen coming in and out of the shot, cleaning the table and placing the objects (bandages, syringes, medical tape, blood pressure machine, etc.).*

*When the live feed begins, we are in* LEAH's *living room. She sits in a red chair by a large window. Next to her is her dialysis machine: a white square piece of machinery, with several saline bags hung above, and threads of plastic medical tubing. On the other side of her is the small wheeled table covered in medical supplies: bandages, medical tape, needles in packages, syringes.*

*She stares down the barrel of the camera for a moment, then speaks.*


LEAH: When I was nineteen I wanted to go to Uganda. I still had my working transplanted kidney back then. My transplant doctor, Dr. Henry Gault, refused to sign my passport application.

> LEAH *picks up a large syringe. We see it has tiny glasses and a lab coat affixed to it. She holds it up and puppets it as Dr. Gault.*

DR. GAULT: Uganda!
I thought your dad and mom were home now.
They've gone again, have they?
Well, Leah, you see . . .

... your creatinine is good. Your blood pressure is slightly elevated, but that's the prednisone, we'd expect that ...
We have had trouble with your transplant. It's stable now.
... but your immune system is compromised.
What about your bloodwork? Who's going to do your bloodwork?
What if you get sick?
Can't you go somewhere else? Go to Halifax. PEI is nice.

LEAH *brings her face down to meet Dr. Gault.*

LEAH: I need to go to AFRICA, Dr. Gault. I can't keep saying no to things because of what might happen, out of fear, right?

*Thoughtful pause.*

DR. GAULT: Well, what am I supposed to say to that?

LEAH *and* DR. GAULT *look at each other.*

*Pause on this. Then* LEAH *lays down the syringe and looks at us.*

LEAH: Good evening folks and welcome. Welcome to *The Dialysis Project.* I can't see you in person but I'm sure I know some of you, and I'm sure you're a lovely crowd.

I'm Leah. I am an actor, obviously, a therapist with a background in psychology. I am also a dialysis patient, and I have been *forever.* Well, not forever. I have had two kidney transplants: one at six years old and a second at eleven years old. The second one lasted twenty-three years, which is considered a success in the transplant world, especially back then. But in 2009 my transplant finally failed and I had to go back on dialysis.

This is my dialysis machine.

*She indicates the machine beside her.*

LEAH: It does two important things for me that your kidneys do for you. Number one, it cleans my blood and, number two, it removes excess fluid.

It pees for me. What you'd pee out, the machine drains out . . . in fact, I never pee otherwise. On a road trip, you'd have to remind me to stop, because unless I need gas or a coffee, I'm likely to just keep going.

I have been on dialysis now for 12 years. I do a treatment every other day. That's a treatment every 48 hours, which works out to over 2,100 treatments, about 4 hours per treatment . . . or a conservative estimate of 8,500 hours on the machine. That's roughly the same amount of time you spent in class in grades one through nine . . . if you didn't miss a day.

Now, even though the treatment takes 4 hours, don't worry: the show won't be that long.

That's right. Tonight I will be actually dialyzing.

There will be medical equipment, and there will be needling in the show; blood will be visible. Just letting you know, in case you have a squeamish side. At least with a livestream there's no "splash zone."

*Short pause.*

This is my house. My home. In downtown St. John's, in the province of Newfoundland and Labrador, the ancestral home of the Beothuk and the Mi'kmaq on the island of

Newfoundland, and the Inuit and Innu of the great land of Labrador.

I dialyze here in my home. Most dialysis patients go to an outpatient unit, full of dialysis chairs. I think the big unit here has 36 seats. Mostly older patients, seniors. All of us just on display, surrounded by buzzing and beeping alarms, nurse chatter.

I learned to self-administer dialysis 10 years ago. Now I do this at home. Every other day. Usually I'm alone. I mean, except for when I'm dialyzing as part of a livestreaming theatre show. And then my stage manager is with me.

Say hi, Jana!

*Her stage manager, Jana, says hello from off camera.*

*Little pause.*

I'm doing this because . . . I want dialysis to be seen, to be witnessed.

Dialysis is probably one of the least talked about—yet one of the most common—chronic procedures. And it is growing in prevalence. It happens every hour, every day. It's happening right now, routine, as routine as a daily shower, if showers took four hours.

*Pause.*

Excuse me for a moment. I've gotta get my snack.

*She gets up and leaves frame, speaks from off camera.*

The thing about dialysis is that it ties you down. When you're reliant upon something like this machine, you can only wander so far—you can't really get too far. You can't fly down to New York City for a weekend, you can't hop over to England to visit friends or jump on a seat sale to Mexico. I often wonder when I watch that old episode of *Grey's Anatomy*—the one with the plane crash and Meredith and Derek and what's-her-bake that Sandra Oh plays . . . they get caught in the middle of the woods and have to keep warm, build a fire until they're rescued.

*She returns and sits.*

I think: I guess there are no dialysis patients in that group . . . two weeks without a treatment, they'd be dead by now.

*She holds up her snacks.*

My snack.

*Beat.*

I've been on the kidney transplant list on and off for twelve years.

I'm what is called "hyper-sensitized" . . . and no, it has nothing to do with being emotional, or being hysterical or prone to hyperbole. It means I have so many antibodies in my blood that finding a kidney match that won't reject is almost impossible.

*Beat.*

This tube-y thing is my kidney now.

*She points to it, connected to the top of the machine, with tubing entering and exiting it.*

It contains a bunch of stringy microfibres—they look like rice vermicelli—the blood pushes through it constantly, over and over again. Tonight, five full litres of blood will exit my body, cycle through 10 feet of medical-grade tubing and this filter and return. Over and over. Twelve full times in all, in one single treatment.

You can't do dialysis just by sticking a needle in your arm. Because all of my blood has to filter through multiple times, they have to surgically create a dialysis site on my body; mine is here in my leg, where I hook up to the machine. They make the site by attaching an artery to a vein, and that creates a really stable and robust blood flow, enough so that two needles can be inserted simultaneously.

One needle for the A, the arterial, where the blood exits the body, and one for the V, or venous, where it pumps back in.

*She pulls her procedure table in front of her, covered in medical tape, bandages, packaged syringes, and needles.*

These are the needles.

*She picks one of them up.*

Dialysis needles are large. You can look through it like a telescope.

*She does.*

You know, when I was training for this, the very first week my nurse was showing me how to needle—I remember turning away from the sight of it. My guts couldn't tolerate the sight of needle breaking skin . . . and I remember my nurse said, "Well, Leah, if you can't even look while we're doing it, you might as well pack up and go home."

She was right. You can't do this without tolerating it . . . but I get it if you don't. If you feel light-headed, you can look away. Lie down, keep a pillow nearby.

I'm gonna start.

> *She begins the needling process. A camera gives us a close-up view of her upper thigh and the dialysis site there.*

First step—clean the site. This is important. I'm going to start with the V-side here. Alright, give it a little wipe. Then we dry it off.

> *She fans the site to dry it while giving us a nonchalant smile.*

Alright, I think we're ready to start with the V. We start with the V because—for you squeamish types, this might be hard to hear—the V is deeper down under the skin and it's just a little bit trickier to needle, so I always start with the tricky one first.

> *Silent concentration for a moment as she inserts the needle. She uses the attached syringe to pull blood to ensure a good flow. She is very practised at this.*

There we go. That was a very smooth needle, for those who are watching. Beauty. That's some good flow. Very easy. The thing I look for when I needle is that the blood flow, coming in and out, is very easy. Smooth. Because this is the needle where the blood is going to push back into my body, and I don't want any resistance or pressure there. So I test it over and over again. I probably test it more than a nurse would.

Now, off we go to the A. It's just the same stuff all over again. Give it a little wipe, make sure it's clean. And dry!

*A brief pause and smile as she fans again.*

Usually doesn't take very long. The cleaning solution is called chlorhexidine. You may have noticed that the A needle is shorter than the V. This is because the A is more superficial, or closer to the skin surface, and much easier to needle. There's always a little blood that appears, so there may be a little squeam on the go. This might be pillow time.

The A is always pretty easy—if you do it every other day. Give it a little try. Whoop. Lovely. Nice, beautiful flow.

Now I'll anchor this baby down with tape so she don't go nowhere. 'Scuse me, I'm showing you my thigh. I'll give it another test because "Leah is persnickety."

There we go. Beauty.

*She looks back to us.*

So how's everyone doing? Still with us? A friend of mine fainted once, watching this. Out like a light. So I just wanted to check in.

So, now I have to hook myself up, but if you have any questions about what I've said so far or what I'm doing, fire away in the chat and I'll get back to you in a bit.

*She begins connecting the tubes.*

I know in most shows they ask you to shut your phone off and put it away. But I'm going to ask you to take yours out. I want you to take them out now.

And I want you to go into your clock and set your timer for 4 hours. Don't press go yet. Wait for me.

Everyone got that done.

Okay, ready to start your timer? Annnnd go.

> *She pushes a button to start her machine. It whirrs and purrs and clicks.*

Okay, you can put your phones away now.

What you are looking at now is the machine filling with my blood.

> LEAH *begins adjusting things on her machine. We see close-up video of her blood moving through the tubes and the filter as she talks.*

> LEAH *moves the table back into side position. She sits back and reclines her chair.*

Okay, let's see if we have any questions.

> *She picks up her computer and accesses the live chat and selects some questions.*

"Does your machine make that noise for the entire treatment?"

Yeah. You get used to it.

"How big is your kidney?"

A real kidney is about the size of your fist.

> *She demonstrates, balling her fist and showing it to the camera.*

"Does it hurt?"

Well the needles don't tickle . . . but after that the treatment doesn't hurt.

"Do a lot of people know you do dialysis?"

> *Beat.*

Well, I used to be pretty private about it.

Now it's mostly a question of when and how I tell someone. Like if you're dating someone new, when do you tell someone you're dating about dialysis? First date? Third date?

Job to say. The bigger question, to be honest, is actually how do you say it?

"Hey, want to come back to my place? I have . . . a machine . . . in my living room."

Sometimes I just fly through the telling really quickly, camouflaging it among other thing: "I'm a Cancer, I love weekends around the bay, I could squish the shit out of a puppy, I self-administer a life-maintaining treatment four times a week, and sushi is one of my favourite foods!"

The truth is that the less I'm into someone, the less I care. The more I'm into someone, the less I want them to know.

*Pause.*

I have a machine in my living room.

I have a walk-in closet blocked with medical supplies.

I have scars, I have a number of surgical scars . . .

*Pause.*

She decides not to pursue this topic right now, decides to take a different direction.

I have a dog.

For most of my life, I had a dog.

My first family pet was Lancer.

I was a toddler when we had him. Lancer was a hunting dog; Dad would take him to the barrens to hunt partridge.

*She takes up some photos off her table, peruses them.*

I remember him, but I wonder how accurate my memories are, because truly my memories of him stem from family photos.

*She shows us a photo of Lancer.*

He was killed on the Trans-Canada when I was four.

Lancer the Second I remember more clearly. We still had Lancer the Second when I had my first transplant when I was six and a half years old.

*She shows us a picture of Lancer the Second.*

I remember thinking about him when I was in the hospital in Toronto, wondering if he'd remember me when I came home. Of course, he always did. Lancer the Second was also killed on the TCH. You'd think we'd have learned to buy a leash. Needless to say, we never named a dog Lancer again.

Sparky came along when I was nine years old.

*She shows us a picture of Sparky.*

I bugged the daylights out of my parents that I wanted a dog, that I was old enough, responsible enough, that I'd walk him and take care of him. I remember the day he arrived. I had counted down the days for weeks and was distracted in class, inattentive. I ran up from the bus stop, and I could hear him from the driveway, yelping. He was in a wooden crate lined with straw, and I went through my dad's tools to find a crowbar to crack him out and set him free, and I tried to walk him on a leash, but he just wanted to sit there and take in his new surroundings.

That transplant kidney rejected two years later, when I was eleven. I did a year of dialysis then, after school on Mondays, Wednesdays, and Fridays, taking the route ten bus to the back entrance of the Health Sciences. I'd be picked up after supper and arrive home around eight p.m. and Sparky would be asleep on my bed, legs in the air and snoring.

One night when I was eleven, at that same dialysis unit, mid-treatment, Dr. Gault stopped at my chair.

*She picks up the Dr. Gault syringe and a smaller one with pigtails. She puppets them as Dr. Gault and a younger version of herself.*

**DR. GAULT**: Leah, if you could have a free flight on the premier's private jet anywhere in the world tonight, where would you go?

**LITTLE LEAH**: To Toronto. For a transplant?

**DR. GAULT**: Well, Leah, tonight is your lucky night.

*Beat.*

**LEAH**: That was midway through grade seven, and I was afraid to leave Sparky—wondered if flying away to Toronto in the middle of the night would confuse him when I wasn't in my room. Transplants don't happen in Newfoundland; adults fly to Halifax and children go to Toronto.

*Pause.*

There were times when I was in Toronto SickKids even before that, when I was really little. There was a woman who worked there and ran the playroom. Her name was Judy.

**JUDY**: Well hello, Leah. I'd love for you to come join us, we have puzzles and little toys and look at that beautiful mural we had painted with all those beautiful little animals on it, do you love animals, Leah? Do you have a little animal at home who's waiting for you?

**LEAH**: Sometimes I would have to be in bed and Judy would come and visit me.

**JUDY**: Well hello, Leah, I thought I would come in a little early and I brought you a book and a puzzle with a silly picture of clowns eating sandwiches at a picnic, Leah, they're having so much fun. Which would you like to do, would you like to put that hard puzzle together, I will help you. Or do you want the book, Leah? Okay.

LEAH *holds up a book.*

JUDY: It's called *Oscar Makes a Friend*, and look at Oscar's little bedroom down in his trash can. Doesn't that look comfortable, Leah? Does that make you think of your bedroom at home, Leah?

Oh, Leah.

Yes, my honey, you're going to go home soon.

Yes, you're gonna see your dog and your little bedroom.

And your mom and dad are going to be there, and they're going to welcome you.

Oh, I know honey. I know.

LEAH *lays the book down.*

*Pause.*

LEAH *motions to the machine.*

LEAH: It's loud, isn't it. This constant annoying hum. Makes it hard to hear the TV, or even my own thoughts sometimes.

Still, doing dialysis at home trumps going to a hospital unit, I can tell you that. I like the privacy and colours of my own space, a familiar space. I decide on what time to hook up and what to watch on TV without negotiating with anyone. I have my own little ice machine that makes little snowy ice cubes shaped like cups, better than the crushed ice at the hospital. I mean, I have to remember to get it before I hook up because once I'm on, there's no one to bring it to me.

I can sit in this nice little recliner I bought online. This one fits me perfectly, I love its shape and colour, it fits perfectly here next to my second-storey window, where I assess the weather and guess the time of day by the approaching dusk.

I love these windows, seeing the green trees of summer, kids idling up the sidewalk with melting ice cream. Autumn and Halloween, my street gets a ton of trick-or-treaters; in December, it's the Mummers Parade. From my window I can sometimes get a view of the action, but I can't really make out what's going on.

    *Pause.*

Dialysis has been around since the late '60s, but it hasn't really changed as a technology. It is essentially the same concept that it was in 1967 or whenever the first dialysis machine was built, which was the size of the wall. This machine is small, but it does the same thing. Replace kidney function. Filter the blood, clean it, remove excess fluid.

In order to connect to the machine, there is the simple necessity of the dialysis site and the ability to maintain it. Everything rides on a functioning site.

I have had seven previous dialysis sites in my life. I've had three in my arms and four in my chest. My current one is in my leg.

*She points to her leg site.*

A leg site is weird because it's pretty rare. Every time I go to the unit, there's always a nurse that's like: "Hey Darlene, come over and watch this little one with the leg graft!"

And then Darlene's like, "Go on, Claudette! Sure, we never see those!"

That's right, you don't see them very often. Because the body only has so many options.

You see, bodies have a love-hate relationship with dialysis. Bodies don't like disruptions, interruptions in the plan as it is laid out. So sites don't last forever. The body fights with them, chokes them out, rejects them. It can happen quickly, it has happened quickly, so I have to check regularly.

*She palpates her site.*

Touch the site, feel the "thrill," the feeling of buzzing that tells you blood is flowing.

Listen to the site.

LEAH *gets a stethoscope and places it on site and listens. We hear what she hears, a rush and whirr.*

Listen for the "bruit"—the word for "sound" in French—a rush like a waterfall that tells you blood is flowing. I analyze the sound; I listen carefully. I listen for its smoothness, confirm it is an uninterrupted pulsating buzz . . . scrutinize with my hearing. Nothing high-pitched, nothing strained, nothing obstructing . . .

*A pause as we listen to the sound and it fades out.*

*She puts the stethoscope away.*

So, online dating. So weird, amiright? I signed up for an online dating site. Long2Belong2009—my profile name.

I hate filling out the profile part, automating what being with someone is supposed to be. Be professional, be athletic. Be a traveller. Looking for dating or long term, looking for friends with benefits, no drama please. No drama? What does that even mean?

I scan through the profiles I look through and feel like I just don't meet the criteria. And honestly, they don't really meet mine either.

What I look for in others, in order to reach out: some sign of a flaw, to be honest. Space. Space for damage . . . or vulnerability . . . and being foolish . . . or something. Room for permission to be damaged too.

I always compare my damaged body to others that aren't— oh my god I do that constantly, all the time. Athletes, mothers giving birth and the fierce energy of motherhood, healthy children starting off with entire able-bodied lives ahead of them, lives that feel on the other side of a pane of glass. I can see it all happening, but I can't get through to join in.

What I want is a sense of belonging, to share a life that isn't compartmentalized by illness.

*Beat.*

So tell me, where does that go in my Long2Belong2009 so that it doesn't send everyone off running, screaming "for the love of god give that one a wide berth!"

*Pause.*

My dog, Sparky, died when I was 24. I was well into my second transplant by then. He was old for a setter. I cried for months—a deep grief that pulled me back to being a kid again. We pulled him in a procession on a red camping sleigh across Little Triangle Pond two days before Christmas. Broke the ground and buried him in the woods. And didn't have another dog for two years.

*Beat.*

Until Fogo.

I remember we picked Fogo up very early one August morning. We laid claim to him over the phone. Me and Flora drove to Carbonear at the break of dawn. He cried himself to sleep on the two-hour drive home, frightened of the new smells, I guess, pink freckled belly facing up . . . his anxiety exhausted him. I slept with him on our den couch for three nights so he'd learn my smell and attach.

Fogo was ten when my second transplant failed. I was about to move to Montreal to do my PhD. I had just turned 35, and I felt a defining line emerge and I began to mark life events as "before" dialysis or "after."

*Footage of her machine begins to play, the voyage of the blood through tubing, the drip of saline in the IV.*

Doing dialysis again was a pain, and exhausting. The unit in Montreal was impersonal and large. My brother called it my part-time job—and all I could think was Gotta get out of this place. Gotta be home to keep Fogo company. After I trained to do my own treatments, Fogo would sleep at the foot of my bed as I prepped my home machine, following me around as I fetched supplies in the laundry room, plopping on his dog bed nearby to settle in for the treatment. It was like he understood we were in for a long haul.

*Footage of machine fades away.*

Fogo died six years ago. He was sixteen. I had to put him down just days before I was scheduled to drive back to Montreal. I made the decision partly because I owed it to him to be buried in Newfoundland, at the foot of our summer place in Holyrood. My dad fixed a plaque to the rock covering his grave. It reads: "Here lies Fogo, lifetime companion."

*Beat.*

LEAH *looks out her window.*

After Fogo, I wasn't sure I'd ever get another dog. Life was a bit of a roller coaster back then dialysis-wise, a lot of unexpected hospital visits. Eighteen invasive procedures for my dialysis site.

Dogs require attention and time—they're basically a 15-year commitment. So . . .

*Pause.*

LEAH *takes off her glasses, rubs her eyes.*

Is this boring? This must be boring.

I'm not used to having people watch this.

I've always felt private about it, dialysis. Secretive. Didn't tell my co-workers.

I guess they know now, hey?

When I do this, usually I'm alone. I don't normally do this with so many people watching. Whose life is so empty and meaningless they got the time to sit and watch someone do dialysis?

No offence.

I know. I know I said I want dialysis to be seen, to be witnessed. But honestly, I actually have grown to resist company when I'm on the machine or at a medical appointment. I'm so used to doing it by myself, being alone for the four hours, that I've settled into a kind of contentment around it. It takes too much energy to be with people; all I want to do is get lost in my own thoughts, watch TV or read a novel, and when I'm with other people I have to expend all this energy to keep up conversation. Sometimes it's stuff I don't even want to talk about. It's kind of awful to admit.

*Pause.*

*A text message pops up on* LEAH's *phone.*

Oh fuck it's this guy again.

Nice enough fella. But a second date is not in the cards.

When he first asked me out, I took three days to answer. Not that he realized it, but he kept suggesting dialysis nights.

We finally agreed on Saturday afternoon. And do you know the first question he asks, like right out of the box? "What makes you happy?"

What makes me happy?

Well that's quite a starter.

Without waiting for my answer, he begins to rattle on about his new SUV: "A base model off the lot, but it still has heated seats. Heated seats are base nowadays."

He's going on about how happy his Kia Sorento makes him for twenty minutes and I'm there thinking, what *does* make me happy?

    *Beat.*

It doesn't take much, as of late. The fall, the grey days when there's no wind or even sun, but the mist on my face feels like a kiss, a light kiss.

A strong, really strong cup of coffee at seven in the morning, my favourite time of day. The company of someone who knows me so well there are no words necessary. Just sitting quietly side by side with our book or our thoughts. Walking, long walks through the downtown, checking out shop windows and thinking. Weekends out of town, berry-picking for hours and bringing home a bucket of berries. A bay house with a view of the ocean from the front window. And humming to myself.

LEAH *hums quietly to herself for a moment.*

*Pause.*

When I was 24 I was living in Montreal going to theatre school—a time when this part of me was kept in a box and none of my friends knew it—a classmate invited me to a family birthday party. Music and dancing and a buffet of homemade food. A woman approached me as I sat on my own watching a network of set dancers doing Through the Woods.

JUDY: Are you Leah? I don't know if you remember me, but I remember you . . . when you were really little. Four, maybe five? You usually played by yourself. I ran the playroom on the 5D ward. I'm Judy.

LEAH: A flush of heat spreads through me. An explosion of emotion. It's not fear, not really, but I do want to escape, find a safe place. I want to go home and sleep, surrounded by warm colours.

*Oscar Makes a Friend.* And the clown picnic.

JUDY: *Oscar Makes a Friend.* The clown picnic. Oh, Leah. That was a hard puzzle, wasn't it?

LEAH: Yes. That was a hard puzzle.

*Beat.*

You know, when I tell stories about dialysis, even now. I feel like I'm in the middle of an uninhabited place, standing at a crossroads. On one hand I want dialysis to be seen and witnessed; I do. On the other, I reject the identity of it.

There's always a part of me that wonders about being at SickKids. A lot went down at SickKids, and we're not going to talk about that today, but sometimes I wonder if it was all just a dream. A part of me doesn't want to believe that it actually happened.

But Judy was there. She saw it happen. I'm not making it up. There were witnesses.

*Pause.*

*She picks up the large Dr. Gault syringe and looks at it.*

Dr. Gault died in 2003. The College of Physicians asked me to write a tribute to him. He was famous in the world of nephrology and dialysis, the inventor of the Cockcroft-Gault formula, a calculation for kidney functioning that is used globally. He was more of a researcher than a teacher, apparently a terrible lecturer. I doubt that was his interest anyway. He was most interested in his patients.

He must have had thousands of patients, easily thousands. But they asked me to write a tribute. I didn't even question it. I knew why: I was his youngest patient; he saw me grow up, he worried when I travelled overseas, he . . . suffered when my first transplant failed, and there was a twinkle in his eye when the call came five years later that another match was found. He wanted to tell me himself. He wanted to deliver the news.

When I heard the news he'd died, I cried. It was like losing a grandfather.

LEAH *puppets the syringe once more.*

DR. GAULT: Thank you for your tribute.

LEAH: You've been gone since 2003.

DR. GAULT: Is it that long?

LEAH: Yes, I remember. Dad called me when I was studying in Vancouver. He told me it was peaceful.

DR. GAULT: Strokes aren't always peaceful. But yes. It was quiet. I was ready.

LEAH: I'm back on dialysis.

DR. GAULT: Yes, we knew that would happen eventually. I'm sorry, Leah.

LEAH: I wanted to tell you . . . I got my PhD. It was rough at times, but worth it.

DR. GAULT: Leah, I'm not surprised. As you always said, you can't say no to things because of what might happen, because of fear, right?

*Pause.*

LEAH *puts down the syringe. Takes a deep breath.*

LEAH: I have a machine in my living room.

I have a walk-in closet blocked with medical supplies.

I have scars.

I have surgical scars on various parts of my body, my neck,

chest, stomach, legs . . . I struggle with loving them, laying claim to the art of them, finding them sexy.

*Pause.*

I step in the door and am welcomed.

"Hey there, beautiful, you've finally decided to come."

Candy, a woman I've met a half-dozen times. I'm wearing a black corset and jeans; I'm terribly, vomitously self-conscious, but have been told by my friends that I look hot.

The party is divided into rooms. Two are reserved for women only. I make my way through the living room: two men, and one is flogging the other with a leather strap, stopping to gently touch the redness between efforts. It's a performance, just as much as it is entirely private . . . couples watch, men, women. Some are intrigued, some turned on, others chat socially: new jobs and summer vacation plans. An ex passes by, a friendly, somewhat awkward exchange—he'd asked me a few times to come to one of these; I'd always said no. He moves on to one of the small rooms in the back: needle play. Not my bag, I think, I have enough needle play in my life already.

I resist the urge to turn around and go home, back to my cat and duvet. I don't want to run away. I keep going, venturing towards the women's space—it's quieter, calmer. Safe . . . I suddenly realize safety is a priority.

I've come here to challenge myself, to explore. I've come here to locate something within me that has been misplaced, replaced instead by procedures and cut skin, where touch has been detached and cold, medical and clinical . . . but still has been more familiar than any other touch.

I watch through the door. I can see Candy inside chatting quietly with a brunette in a leather jacket. They both turn and notice me, and Candy smiles.

"Come sit with us," she says.

I squeeze in beside her . . .

Candy touches my arm. "It's just about to start."

The performer makes her way into the little open space, lit with a red house lamp. It's breezy and sensual, like a warm August afternoon before a rainstorm. She begins to move rhythmically and a dance emerges, her back curling like a cat's. She turns away from us, releasing her blouse to the floor; all eyes follow her and will her to turn around, and I catch a glimpse of what looks familiar. Is that . . . ?

A surgical scar peeking out from under her arm.

She turns to face us, a cross-section line across a flattened chest. Bilateral mastectomy. Skipping reconstruction, opting instead for a ring of wildflowers running diagonally across her whitened scar and ending below her left shoulder.

Candy says: "Gorgeous, eh?"

Pause.

And I think: Gorgeous?

Yes, gorgeous.

This body. My body. Uniquely cut out and unlike any other—uneven skin and pinkness of scars. This body is bumped and bruised and pricked and cut with scars that rise up above the skin and call out, drawing attention to other things that are both beautiful and ugly—simultaneously.

The ugly part is about brokenness, new marks that are revealed when clothing falls away—when someone looks at me naked—nausea from fear, held breath—I expect shock and am prepared. This is me. You can see it now—I'm inviting you in if you want.

This. Is. Me.

I'll accept if you gasp, if you walk away. Prepared for rejection, repulsion, deem it something you don't want. The ugly part has to do with cuts and puffiness and fantasizing about a trade-in.

The beauty part is about confidence and touch and sex and feeling desired. They don't reject. They aren't repelled or made sick or frightened off. They are pulled in. Drawn close.

They touch.
They kiss.
They smile.

And return. They come back again . . .

The beauty comes from that shock—and it heals me. A shock that heals . . . happy to be seen naked then—this body can do that—this body can.

>	*Beat.*

I stayed on at the party later than I'd planned, arrived back at my apartment sometime after five, somehow not alone. "Mind if we crash?" My ex from earlier.

And a friend.

And I say yes.

And I know what "Mind if I crash, missed my ride" means. But it's really fine, though . . . It's actually soft and easy, safe and warm. Bodies entangled. What would have frightened, even paralyzed me before, now feels safe and protected. We sleep then, a thunderstorm welling through the open window.

> *Thunder sound in the distance and then louder. Then louder. Suddenly what was beautiful is ominous.*

> *A video plays:* LEAH *in hospital in a candid conversation with an ER doctor. It is a real clip of* LEAH *seeking emergency care for the dialysis site in her arm, which is in crisis. The doctor talks* LEAH *through the options for her care, including putting a stent in her arm site as a last-resort measure to salvage it. She looks stressed and scared. After it ends:*

LEAH: That doctor did put a stent in my arm. It's right here. But it didn't work.

My dialysis site is now in my leg. As you know.

> *Beat.*

A leg site is so unusual that two other surgeons wouldn't even consider it. But my surgeon went for it because . . . well, it was the only option.

Having a site in your leg essentially means your upper body has become uncooperative with dialysis, offering no more viable site options.

There are limited options in both legs . . . so we work hard to keep this one pumping.

Walking.
Fish oil.

I'm not even sure I can make a difference; I get mixed messages. The dialysis folks say, "Yes, keep your BP up, keep the blood moving." The vascular surgeons say, "Naw, there's nothing you can do to prevent it from blocking. It's not your fault . . ."

My nurse calls my dialysis site my "lifeline," and she's right. My site has to work in order for dialysis to happen. If a site stops working and another one can't be created within 72 hours, then . . . When you no longer have options for dialysis sites, you can't do dialysis, and if you can't do dialysis, then you'll die within a matter of weeks.

   *Beat.*

I know my friends worry. I realize it's been difficult for them, a struggle to stay, to sit with me. That time Cherie filmed me in hospital. The many times I've texted Willow or Danielle on the way to Emerge at 3 a.m. When Robert and Di intervened with that nurse. She didn't have a clue, she kept asking the same line of questions over and over and lost patience with my upset and Di and Robert raised their voices, pleading to just listen. Listen to her.

Sit with me in my fear.

Waking in the wee hours by myself. Automatically checking that my site is still buzzing, still whirring away. Listening for the bruit. That rush like a waterfall that tells you blood is flowing. The fear of touching and feeling nothing. Hearing no bruit.

I've been there. Calling and reporting to the hospital switchboard. A strange voice at the end of the phone. "Okay my love, I'll get the doctor on the line . . . just hold for a second okay?" . . . Time ticking by, seconds into minutes, minutes into hours, hours into days . . . "I'm going to need another treatment by tomorrow morning." This might be the time where they won't save it, they won't be able to keep it flowing . . . and they won't get it clear.

"I think your site must have blocked out on us again, Leah."

LEAH *takes a deep breath.*

Calm down.

If I'm upset, I'll be dismissed . . . if I'm stressed, I won't be listened to. It happens in hospitals sometimes, when lives get challenged by illness . . . the assumption that hospitals are unfamiliar and can't be navigated, so medical teams say give them space, give them time to calm down.

But I know hospitals like I know my own fucking living room . . . I know this shit like the back of my hand. I don't want, I don't need space to calm down . . . I just need someone to see it, to know what I know, and to say: "Yes, this is serious, yes we need to act on this, yes . . . you're right, Leah, this is vital. This is important. We got you, Leah."

And when that's missed, when what I know, know as clearly as the chair I'm sitting in, when that is pushed aside, that fear shifts to rage.

Then I have to work hard at grounding myself, at organizing my words, then I have to redirect my energy. And I have to take charge. I'm the one who has to take charge. No one else is going to do it. I'm the one.

I had to make discoveries within the system in order to optimize the care of my site. I had to be like a broken fucking record in order to get there

The doctor is trying to calm me down by being dismissive: "I think your site must have blocked out on us again, Leah."

I'm like, fuck you, it's not "us," it's me! It's not fucking "us"!

This is me!

*A silence.*

LEAH *takes off her glasses, rubs her eyes.*

*She slowly recovers.*

*Eventually:*

Sometimes I dream impossible things.

A dream that's come and gone since I was four . . . I can fly . . .

*A video fades in. An animated skyline, birds and clouds.*
*An animated figure that might be* LEAH *twists and tumbles*
*in the sky. The video plays throughout the following.*

Eyes closed, one two three . . . I fill my lungs, they fill with
ease and send a shot of energy through my body; I move
my arms and my strength lifts my weight and I can, yes
I can. I can. With a running start, I leap and am airborne.
And with only my will, I begin to float:

A shriek of laughter, I'm surprised at my strength; my
muscles are alive, my legs can work hard. I want to rise
higher, to a higher point. Out the door and down the
street, zipping past my pacing neighbour and local tomcat
perched on the back fence, I whir past Holy Heart school
and the skating arena with its year-round snow hill. I smile
and wave, what a beautiful day isn't it? The wind is cold on
my face, but the sun is warm on my body. I don't need a
sweater or a jacket.

The higher I climb, the stronger I feel.

I fly downtown, and bang on Robert's door. Come out.
Come fly with me . . . we make our way up Signal Hill—
I show him how—the fall colours glowing.

We drop by Flora's house and pull her out too . . . I make
my rounds and grab everyone and make them float too,
'cuz my power is so strong I can give it away . . . Willow
and Dave and Roxy, and Diana, and Danielle and . . . and
gather them all, and we go.

We take flight together. We rise above the clouds and

laugh out loud at the vastness of it all. The treetops over Bannerman and Bowring parks, the rocky barrens and the berry pickers, the harsh vastness of the Northern Peninsula, we drop down and pick up Didi—the island of Newfoundland grows small and falls away as we again gain a tremendous height . . . we fly to Montreal and Toronto, collect Evalyn, Caroline and Gerard and Melissa and Cherie.

We head to New York and perch on the crown of the Statue of Liberty. We sip on americanos and nibble soft pretzels, then head on over to San Francisco and visit the Golden Gate Bridge. We go to the Grand Canyon, the Great Wall of China, the pyramids. I feel the crisp wind against my cheeks.

*The dream and video are interrupted by an abrupt alarm.*

LEAH *who had been gazing out the window, looks to her machine. She presses a button.*

Three more hours.

*A long pause.*

LEAH *indicates her leg site.*

This site has blocked three times in the last year.

Dialysis sites last three to five years and this one is in its fifth year now.

I've been told that I have one option left, in my right leg, which is supposed to last the rest of my life.

I've always had this notion in the back of my head that eventually medicine would figure something out, or that the phone would ring with news of a transplant . . . and pretty much every other time that has been true. But this is complicated. This is even out of medicine's hands in many ways.

*Silence.*

So much has happened.

So much is happening and there is so much more to say that isn't about the dialysis, that relegates dialysis to being that annoying hum in the background.

And sometimes it's about what you grab onto while the hum hums on.

I've grabbed onto a lot.

I have a house.

I have friends.

I have close friends and not-so-close friends.

I have family.

I have cousins who are friends.

I have nurses who know me well, who compare me to their sister, their daughter, their friend.

I have nurses to go to battle for me sometimes. Who speak for me when the doctors don't get it.

I have a voice, not all the time, but I use it when I need to.

I have a new dog. Her name is Bea.

I have a machine in my living room.

I have a walk-in closet blocked with medical supplies.

I have surgical scars on various parts of my body, my neck, chest, stomach, legs.

I have a heavy pulsation of blood whirring through my left thigh. Just my left, not the right. The right is silent and still. For now.

I have laughter that's sometimes uncontrolled and face pinching. Breathless, squeaking laughter when no one else finds it funny.

I have light through this window.

I have access to the early morning, the sun cresting the Narrows and being smacked by the sight of it.

I have a chair on a deck with a view of the ocean.

I have a PhD.

I have dreams where I can fly.

I have hope.

    *Beat.*

Actually scratch that.

I have fear.

I have confusion.

I have rage.

But I have agency.

And that's going to work for me when I need it to.

And when they see me coming, they see it.

I have moments where I feel alone.

But I also know that I have a shared story. Whether you live on dialysis or with an insulin pump or if you've rung the chemo bell or live with daily pain. Whether you're the one on the gurney or the one who sits in the waiting room—there are pieces of my story that don't apply to you, I know that—it doesn't matter, that doesn't matter.

I think what does matter is that the hum in the background, whatever it may be, however loud, or deafening, what matters is that hum does not take over, doesn't define us as people. People with lives and loves and animal connections . . . people that refuse to get lost in the secrecy. People that are not alone. Even though we may sit solitary in our chairs.

    *Beat.*

So . . . I'm going to sit a bit longer in this one. Thanks for coming tonight. It means a lot.

    *She looks out the window.*

    *The video feed fades away.*

**THE END**

# ACKNOWLEDGEMENTS

The creators of *The Dialysis Project* would like to thank the following for making it all possible:

Buddies in Bad Times Theatre; Mel Hague; Sarah Garton Stanley; The National Arts Centre Collaborations, Morgan Jones Phillips; Erin Brubacher; Brad Hart; Blair Voyvodic; Suzanne Robertson and Fox; Diana Daly; Flora Planchat; Luke Dobson; Lori Clarke; Lois Brown; David and Karen Hood; the Admiralty House Museum; Willow and Dave Jackson-Anderson; Roxy Jackson-Anderson; Bryar Smith; Glenn Nuotio; Erin Holland; Sharon MacDonald and the Home Dialysis Program at Eastern Health; MUN Research Team: Jan Buley, Natalie Beausoleil, Pam Ward, Abdullah Saif (Doctoral Student, Community Health); MUN Research Centre for the Study of Music, Media, and Place; the auto-ethnography research writing group at MUN; Faculty of Education's Writing Group.

LEAH LEWIS
Creator/Writer/Performer

Leah Lewis is an artist and scholar. She has worked as an actor and writer within the provincial arts industry for many years, with theatre, film and television credits that include Artistic Fraud's adaptation of Michael Crummey's work *Salvage: The Story of a House*, Pope Productions' adaptation of Ed Riche's *Rare Birds*, and others. Leah merges her love of the arts with her research in her assistant professor position with Memorial University's Faculty of Education's Counselling Psychology graduate program. In particular, Leah applies the arts to research that considers the patient's role and input to health outcomes. *The Dialysis Project* is the second in a series of Leah's arts-based work on patient voice and health.

## EVALYN PARRY
Creator/Director

Evalyn Parry is a multi-disciplinary theatre-maker: director, writer, songwriter, performer, and collaborator committed to performance that invites challenging conversations, and personal and social transformation. From 2015 to 2020, she served as artistic director of Buddies in Bad Times Theatre in Toronto. Parry's genre-defying works *Kiinalik: These Sharp Tools* and *SPIN* have toured nationally and internationally; other notable productions include *Obaaberima* by Tawiah M'Carthy (Buddies; Dora Award for Outstanding Production), *Gertrude and Alice* (Buddies / Independent Aunties; Governor General's Literary Award nominee) and the acclaimed queer, intergenerational *Youth / Elders Project* (Buddies). Evalyn is the recipient of numerous Dora Mavor Moore Awards, as well as the K. M. Hunter Award for Theatre and the Ken McDougall Award for Directing; she has also released five albums of original music. www.evalynparry.com

ROBERT CHAFE
Creator/Dramaturge

Robert Chafe has worked in theatre, dance, opera, radio,
fiction, and film. His stage plays have been seen in Canada,
the United Kingdom, Australia, and the United States; they
include *Oil and Water*, *Tempting Providence*, *Afterimage*,
*Under Wraps*, *Between Breaths*, *Everybody Just C@lm the
F#ck Down*, and *The Colony of Unrequited Dreams* (adapted
from the novel by Wayne Johnston). He has been short-
listed twice for the Governor General's Literary Award for
drama, and he won the award for *Afterimage* in 2010.
He has been guest instructor at Memorial University,
Sir Wilfred Grenfell College, and the National Theatre
School of Canada. In 2018 he was awarded an honorary
doctorate from Memorial University. He is the playwright
and artistic director of Artistic Fraud.